Understanding YOUR Skin

Discover The Foundations of Skincare from Understanding Your Skin Type and Identifying Common Skin Concerns to Building a Personalized Skincare Routine That Caters to Your Unique Needs.

Your Ultimate Guide to Healthy - Radiant And Glowing Skin

NDAHAFA MUTONGOLUME

CONTENTS

INTRODUCTION 1

CHAPTER 1: How Does The Skin Function? 7

CHAPTER 2: What Is Your Skin Type? 15

CHAPTER 3: Skin Condition 19

CHAPTER 4: Skincare Routine 24

CHAPTER 5: Skin Treatment 30

CHAPTER 6: Key Ingredients.. 35

CHAPTER 7: Skin & Diet.. 63

Introduction

The secret to healthy, happy skin lies in understanding your skin.

I know firsthand how hard it can be to find the perfect product regime that works for you because I have battled with numerous skin issues over the years. I am here to discuss the value of understanding the skin and how to improve your skincare regimen. Our skin is the largest organ in the human body and our first line of faded face in the outer world. It protects us from pollutants, skin harming, UV radiation and other environmental dangers. Nevertheless, not all our skin is created equal. Everybody's skin is unique and needs and concerns. Understanding your skin is therefore crucial to having excellent skin. Knowing your skin type, problems, and needs will help you select the best products and regimes for you.

There is a skincare routine out there that will work wonders for you regardless of whether you have oily, dry, sensitive or mixed skin; and understand your skin. Understanding your skin implies being aware of your skin type, issues and requirements, oily, dry, combination, and sensitive skin are the four main types. You can identify your skin type by looking at the unique traits of each skin type; for instance, dry skin can feel tight and scratchy and be prone to fine lines and wrinkles. Oily skin often produces excessive oil and is prone to acne. The first step in knowing your skin is to identify your skin type. To do this, keep an eye on your skin all day long and know how it feels. The second step is to take a closer look at your pores. Are they big and obvious, or are they tiny barely noticeable? Finally, think about any skin issues you may have, such as acne or sensitivity.

After determining your skin type, it's important to understand your skincare routine may vary as a result, for instance, if you have oily skin, you should use light weight cosmetics that won't clog your pores. On the other hand, you should use hydrating and moisturizing creams. If you have dry skin, you can select the ideal skincare products and regime for you by being aware of your skin type. By doing this, you can prevent or address potential problems and have skin that is healthy and happier.

Understanding your skin type, needs, and concerns has a number of benefits including:

Better product selection: when you know what type of skin you have, you can select skincare products that are effective for you, for instance, you should stay away from heavy or oily creams that can clog your pores if you have oily skin. In its place, you should search for light weight oil free cosmetics that aid in regulating sedum production and avoiding acne. You can get better results and prevent any negative reactions by picking the proper items for your skin type.

Targeted treatments: knowing your skin troubles will help you select your best skin regime and take care of problems, for instance, you should utilize products that contain Vitamin C or Niacinamide serum that can brighten and level out your skin tone if you have hyperpigmentation. You can address your unique challenges and receive greater outcomes by choosing focus therapy.

Increased skin health: you may take better care of your skin and enhance its general health by recognizing your skin type and its requirements. For instance, if you have dry skin, you should use moisturizing and hydrating creams to avoid dryness, fine lines and wrinkles by taking care of your skin requirements, you can shield it from harm and enhance its general health.

Prevent skincare mistakes: by being aware of your skin type, you can prevent typical skincare mistakes, for instance, if you have oily skin in order to prevent adding more oil to your skin to make up for the deficiency in moisture, your skin may end up using extra oil as a result of this you can prevent this mistake and get better outcomes by being aware of your skin type and its requirements.

Save your time and money: knowing your skin can help you maintain better skin health while also saving you time and money over the long run by choosing the proper products and treatments, you can avoid investing in items that are ineffective for your skin type or addressing problems that do not concern you. Understanding your skin type, concerns, and needs is crucial for achieving healthy, happy skin. By choosing the right products and treatments, you can improve your skin's health and prevent any concerns from arising in the future. So take the time to understand your skin and reap the benefits.

Common skincare concerns: now that we have discussed the importance of understanding your skin. Let's talk about some common skincare concerns that people face. These concerns can range from acne, aging, hyperpigmentation, and they can be addressed with the right products and treatments.

Acne is a common worry for many people, and it can be brought on by a number of things, including lifestyle, hormones and avidity. It's essential to use products that are not comedogenic and won't clog your pores. If you have acne-prone skin, finding the right products for your skin type and specific requirements is crucial because what works for one person might not work for another.

Aging: everyone ages naturally, but certain things, such as pollution and sun exposure can speed up the process. It's crucial to use Anti-aging cosmetics with SPF and antioxidants to protect your skin from harm; moreover, search for products containing retinoids which can add in minimizing the appearance of wrinkles and fine lines. Once more, it's crucial to pick items that are suitable for your skin type and specific requirements.

Hyperpigmentation is a disorder in which some areas of the skin become darker than the surrounding skin, sun exposure, acne, and hormone changes are some of the factors that can cause hyperpigmentation. To help lighten and bring out your skin tone, use treatments containing Vitamin C which helps treat hyperpigmentation; of course, there are still so many things to learn about our skin and how to choose the right products and regime, but with the help of resources like this book **UNDERSTANDING YOUR SKIN** you can gain a deeper understanding of your skins unique needs and develop a personalized skincare routine that will work best for you. If you are looking to learn more about your skin and how to care for it, you might find it helpful. The secret to healthy, happy skin lies in understanding your skin by taking the time to identify your skin type, concerns, and needs. You can make better decisions when it comes to choosing the right skincare products and treatments. Let's face it, with so many options out there, choosing the right products can be overwhelming, but understanding your skin can make the process a lot easier and it's not just about choosing the right product. Understanding your skin can also help you avoid common skincare mistakes that can lead to breakouts, irritation and other unpleasant side effects.

By knowing what works for your skin and what doesn't, you can save yourself time, money and frustrations in the long run.

This book is packed with valuable information and insight and not just the proper regime for the skin's need but also on the layers of the skin. Learn how deep down your products penetrate in the skin for it to make a difference and promote healing. You will learn about the skin's barrier, the acid mantle, how to hydrate the skin, and much more.

This book is for every skin type.

Chapter 1

How Does The Skin Function?

The skin is the largest organ of the body. It is an elastic protective covering, which is thinnest on the lips and eyelid and thickest on the palms of the hands and soles of the feet. Understanding how it functions will help you know how products function in the skin, as well as knowing how the aging process starts and how to prevent it.

In this chapter, you will learn about these 4 things that will get you a step closer to having the skin of your dreams.

- Layer of the Skin
- Skin Barrier
- Acid mantle
- How to hydrate the Skin

Layers of the Skin

The skin is made up of three layers:

Epidermis: first layer of our bodies which is continually being regenerated because it is covered by dead cells. They protect the body against the outside world.

Dermis: the second layer made of collagen fibers, they keep the skin strong and flexible.

Hypodermis: third layer which provides backup and support

Epidermis Layer

This is the outermost layer of the skin, which forms a protective covering of the body. Squamous cells are correctional sites produced in the skin's basal layer (see structures of the skin). These cells then migrate up through the epidermis until they complete their life circle and the dead stratum corneum.

The epidermis contains the following 5 layers:

Stratum corneum

This is compost of tightly part dead cells which are constantly being shut and replaced. This layer contains the skin's natural moisturizing factors and is responsible for maintaining the cornified layer's hydration. Natural moisturizer factors exist inside corneocyte.

Stratum lucidum

This layer is a barrier compost of transparent cells through which light can pass. These cells are only presents in thick skins such as the palm of the hands and soles of the feet.

Stratum granulosum

These consist of dying cells that contain distinct granules. They are keratinocytes that migrate from the layers below the spinous layer that are causing granules.

Statum spinosum

Consist of multiple layers of square shaped cells, the desmosomes that hold the cells together have a spiny or prickle like appearance when viewed under a microscope. As cells move upward during natural cell turnover, they become flatter. This layer also contains langer cells that assist in the skin's immune function.

Stratum Basale

These consist of keratinocytes that undergo cell division and are responsible for the growth of the epidermis. These layers also contain melanocytes that protect the cell from the UV rays of the sun. This is where melanin comes from, the build-up of these cells are the factor causing conditions of hypo and hyperpigmentation, melasma and dark spots.

Dermis Layer

The dermis layer is the layer underneath the epidermis. Consisting of highly sensitive and mash connective tissues, collagen, elastin, hyaluronic acid and fibroblast. Once treatments and products reach this layer of the skin, that's when the skin drastically improves.

Hypodermis or subcutaneous layer

This is the fatty layer laying directly below the skin, which is composed of fat cells, blood nerves and limp supply. It gives smoothness and contours to the body. Contains fat that is utilized by the body for energy and acts as a protection for the outer skin.

Skin Barrier

The skin barrier function refers to the strength of the skin barrier and like while it protects the skin from environmental factors. The top layer of the skin stratum corneum resembles a break and modem complex, and it's made up of two components.

The nonliving cells that are ready to shed, the break and lipids which are made up of fats, oils, waxes, hormones and vitamins, are contained in the skin. The lipid barrier helps maintain skin hydration, which contributes to the feeling of soft skin, a healthy lipid barrier traps water in the skin and prevents water loss and the natural moisturizing factors from leaving through the outermost layer of the skin.

The stratum corneum

This term known as trans epidermal water loss, also prevents chemical and biological irritants and the environment from entering into the skin. The environmental factor that affects the health of the lipid barrier are aging, water, too much washing causes loss of natural moisturizing factor in the skin, sun damage from the UV rays, and UVp chemical influences such as detergents solvents and the over use of perfumes. They can alter the skin's natural PH levels and cause the skin to become dry and sensitive. The rise and fall and temperature humidity, for example, cold temperatures cause dehydration and sensitivity in the skin and high humidity can cause an increase in sebum also known as oil production, leaving the skin to be moist and shiny and making sugar condition such as acne or essecia.

The signs that your lipid barriers have been broken.

Dryness, cracked skin, sometimes even bleeds, flaky skin, rough texture and scaly texture. Cosmetics products can restore the natural moisturizing factors in the skin. To maintain the water content and the moisture in the skin.

Adequate hydration of the top layer of the skin maintains the plasticity of the skin and protects it from damage, as well as helping it to shut old cells effectively. Ingredients such as oils and fatty acids form a firm on the surface of the skin to prevent water loss from the top layer of the skin and are great in maintain moister.

Acid mantle

The acid mantle is the thin protective film that sits on the surface of the skin which comes from skin sebum sweats and acts as a barrier between the skin and the outside world. It has a slightly acidic PH level and approximately PH 5.5 but can range from PH 4.5 to PH 6.5. It also depends on your individual skincare chemistry and the kind of products being used on the skin.

What does the acid mantle do?

Barrier function prevents too much trans-epidermal water loss to maintain the skin's normal moisture level and provides protection against pollutants UV rays, and temperature change.

Maintaining the skin's pH balance is important, and maintaining skin's softness, suppleness, smoothness, strength, and resistance to infection provides protection against harmful bacteria and prevent microorganisms from growing. The pH of the acid mantle is acidic as bacteria thrive in alkaline conditions. Boost the immune system by producing antigens close to the surface of the skin so they can kill the bad bacteria.

Factors affecting the acid mantle.

Genetic, aging as the skin becomes drier, products not suiting your skin type, lifestyle such as smoking, diet, air, water, sun pollution. The application of cosmetics and personal care products: detergents such as laundry soaps or cleanser, skin moister, sweat and sebum beauty and chemical treatments.

Characteristics of a disrupted acid mantle.

Skin conditions such as eczema, rosacea and dermatitis, burning, itching or hot feeling sensation on the skin or inflammation, skin prone to scars and other marks, as well as dry, dehydrated skin.

How to protect and restore the acid mantle.

1. Avoid using harsh products that strips your skins natural oils.
2. Us products that are within the skin healthy ph. range, which is the ph. 4.5 to ph. 6.5.
3. Use sunscreen to preserve the acid mantle.
4. Consider what you eat
5. Use oil or jell based cleansers to help restore the skins moister and also to balances oil production.

How to hydrate the skin

The skin looks its best when it is hydrated; it looks more youthful, vibrant and supple appearance and has a down glow. Keeping hydrated both internally and externally to keep it looking its best for years to come.

Internally

Drink water 2 litres to 1 gallon per day diet such as fruits and vegetables.

Externally

Moisturize with a cream or oil such as jojoba oil or sweat almond oil

Gently cleansing products that do not contain harsh ingredients that strip off the skin's natural oils and harm the lipid barrier nor the acid mantle.

Chapter 2

What Is Your Skin Type?

Introduction to skincare

There are 4 common skin types: oily, dry, combination, and sensitive. A skin type is determined by how much or how little oil your skin produces. Genes, diet, stress level, hormonal fluctuation, medication and even your skincare regimen all determine how much oil your skin produces.

For you to determine what your skin type is, it is best to do a skin test. To do this, you must wash your face, pat it dry, then after a few minutes, take a piece of lens cleaning tissue paper and press on different spots on your skin if your skin is oily, the paper will stick. Pick up oil spots and become translucent. If the paper doesn't stick or pick up any oily spots, then it is most likely dry. If the paper sticks to your t-zone (forehead, nose, and chin), then you have normal or combination skin.

Below, you will find a description of each skin type, the symptoms you will experience and what product type to use to bring balance to the skin.

Dry skin type

Symptoms:

- Slight to severe flaking, scaling and peeling
- Cracking
- Itching
- Redness
- Skin appears and feels rough.
- Feeling of tightness after encountering water

Product type:

Use a rich moisturizer; it may be necessary to change your moisturizer according to the different seasons. Use a thicker one in the winter and a thiner one during the summer.

Oily skin type

Symptoms:

- Large pore

- Skin appears shiny or dull.
- Shows an oily residue if blotted with tissue.
- Skin is prone to acne and blemishes.

Product type:

Use liquids such as light gel serums and thin lotions as opposed to thick products that can clog pores. Avoid using products that contain harsh ingredients like alcohol, as it can trigger more oil production and become problematic.

Sensitive skin type:

Symptoms:

- Stinging sensation when using products
- Skin likely to be dry or hyper-reactive(highly sensitive)
- In flamed or irritated
- Shows skin conditions such as eczema, rosacea or allergies
- Maybe red or flush easily

Product type

Avoid products that use fragrance, alcohol or any other harsh ingredients such as AHA, BHA, and Retinol

Combination skin type

Symptoms:

- Oily in the T-zone (forehead, nose, and chin)
- Other parts of the face are dry and flaky or without shine.

Product type

Light weight formulas such as gel liquids and oil absorbing products. Lotions and creams for the dry areas.

Chapter 3

Skin Condition

There are 4 main skin conditions:

- **Acne**
- **Aging**
- **Hyperpigmentation**
- **Sensitive**

Although in the world of skincare, there are 24 different skin conditions. Here is a list of the 24 skin conditions and a brief description of each.

Adult acne

Acne breakouts due to hormonal changes or other factors.

Asphyxiated

Smokers have asphyxiated skin from lack of oxygen. City dwellers are also those that are characterized by clogged pores and wrinkles, dull and lifeless looking, and can be yellowish or grey in color.

Comedones

Open comedones are blackheads and clogged pores caused by buildup of debris, oil and dead skin cells stuck in the pores. The oxidation is what causes it to be dark in color. Closed comedones are not open to the air or oxygen. They are trapped by dead skin cells and need to be exfoliated, and extracted; also called whitehead if hardened.

Couperose

Redness; distended capillaries from weakening of the capillary wall, internal or external causes.

Cyst

Fluids, infection, or other matter under the skin.

Dehydration

Lack of water in the skin. Also caused by the environment i.e., heat, winter, medications, topical agents, aging or dehydrating drinks such as caffeine and alcohol. This can cause the skin to look dull in appearance, discolored and prematurely.

Eczema

Caused by change in season, dehydration, stress and poor digestion just to name a few, it comes out in the form of dry, inflamed or wet eczema.

Enlarge pores

Large pores due to excess oil and debris trapped in the follicles or expansion due to elasticity loss or trauma.

Erythema

Redness caused by inflammation or post extractions or pressure on the skin.

Hyperkeratinization

An excessive buildup of dead skin cells/keratinized cell.

Hyperpigmentation

Brown or dark pigmentation, discoloration from melanin production due to sun, other factors such as hormones, medications or irritation.

Hypopigmentation

White colorless areas from lack of melanin production, cannot be repaired.

Irritation

Usually redness or inflammation from a variety of causes, internal or external

Keratosis/keratoses

A buildup of cells, a rough texture.

Millia

Hardened whitehead oil and dead skin cells trapped beneath the surface of the skin. These are not exposed to oxygen and have to be lanced to open and remove them.

Papules

Raised lesions are also called blemishes.

Poor elasticity

Sagging loose skin from damage, the sun and aging.

Psoriasis

This is a common, chronic genetic systematic inflammatory disease that is characterized by symptoms and signs such as elevated itchy plaques of raised red skin covered with a thick silvery scale. Psoriasis is usually found on the elbows, knees and scalp but can often affect the legs, trunk and nails.

Pustules

An infected papule with fluid inside

Rosacea

A vascular disorder, chronic redness. Papules and pustules may be present

Sensitivities

Reactions from external and/or internal causes. Also named eczema, psoriasis and rosacea.

Solar comedones

Large blackheads, usually around the eyes, due to sun exposure.

Sun damage

UV damage to the epidermis and dermis primary effects are wrinkles, collagen and elastin breakdown, pigmentation and cancer.

Wrinkle/aging

Lines and damage from internal or external causes also expression lines.

Chapter 4

Skincare Routine

Introduction to Skincare Routine

A skincare regimen is essential to beautiful, healthy skin. Once you put your skin on a daily, weekly and monthly routine, your skin will reap the benefits of having healthy, younger looking skin longer.

If any issues or conditions happen to arise through the course of your life due to other contributing factors discussed throughout, having a regular routine for your skin is what will help it return to its natural.

The products in your routine will also change throughout the year, depending on the seasons. During the fall and winter months, the skin tends to be drier and lacking in moisture, so you will want to use creamier cleansers and thicker hydrating creams for both day and night. The spring and summer produce more oils in the skin due to the excessive heat and hot sun. Using lighter gel-like moisturizers and gel or foaming cleansers for a deeper clean is ideal during these months to avoid clogging the pores.

Follow the steps in this weekly skincare routine:

Weekly Skincare Routine

Cleanser (Morning & Night)

Before you begin, remove any make-up with a make-up remover or a deep cleansing oil for the eyes, face and lips. Rinse the skin with water and apply a quarter-type amount of the cleanser that is appropriate for your skin type and condition. In small circular motions, move from the center of the face outward, wash the face thoroughly to remove all dirt or oil and deep rinse the skin with lukewarm water making sure to get all the cleanser from the hairline and jawline.

Toner (Morning & Night)

Toners rinse away traces of oils, fats and residue from cleansers tighten pores, restores the skins pH factor, stimulate circulation and fine texture. After cleansing hold the bottle 12 inches from the face and spray directly on the skin with 4 squads, leave the skin damp to help with hydration and apply the moisturizer on top. Another way for application is to spray the cotton pad directly with the toner and apply it on the face, wiping from the forehead down to the jawline.

Eye cream (Morning & Night)

To reduce puffiness under your eyes circle and close fits, an eye cream is necessary, use half of a pee size and with your two ring fingers, apply the eye cream and accouter clockwise motions, first circular and then a patting motion to awaken the muscle around the eye area.

Serum (Morning & Night)

Serums are highly concentrated and are great home treatments for daily use to help with the improvement and maintenance of your skin. Due to its high concentration of ingredients, 1 to 2 pumps is all you need for the whole face. Wrap the serum in your hands lightly and greatly pat it on the skin, then begin what we call the doctor jack massage to help penetrate the serum into the skin. Gather four fingers and squeeze gently while giving your skin a slight twist or need. The skin needs to be dry before applying moisturizer or facial oil.

Moisturize (Morning)

Moister is different from oil, so even those with the oiliest skin need to moisturize daily. With the appropriate moisturizer for your skin type and up and down and outward motions. Starting from the lower cheeks, then moving to your forehead using upwards strokes, down the temple, down to the nose and then back to the up, down and outwards motion on the cheeks coming around to your chin and jawline and side to side in the sweeping motion. Make sure to use firm pressure to promote proper blood circulation.

SPF (Morning)

No matter what the weather is outside or what the season is SPF should be worn daily. With the same application techniques as the moisturizer, apply the SPF the same way, and SPF is great to be cocktailed with the moisturizer to avoid any white residue left over with the SPF.

Hydrate (Night)

Our skin rejuvenates and heals itself throughout the night. So, hydrating and treating the skin at night is a must to help along with the healing process that the skin naturally does. Use the same application protocol as for the daytime moisturizer for the nighttime hydrating process, and this time, make sure to apply serum and hydrator to your neck and chest and upward strokes towards your jawline.

Exfoliate (Night)

Choose a night in the week to exfoliate the dead cells, build up the breed, and oil up the skin. After cleansing, pat the skin dry and apply the exfoliator in small circular motions all over the face, including the forehead and neck, using medium to firm pressure. Exfoliate the skin for about 2-3 minutes, then rinse with lukewarm to cool water.

Mask (Night)

Mask helps to further treat the skin and leave it looking more youthful and fresher. Pour about 2-3 amount in a small dish on the palm of your hand and apply the mask downward motions all over the face and neck, skipping the eye area. Leave on for 10-20 minutes, then rinse off with warm water; continue the steps for the nighttime routine by applying the serum and hydrator.

Facial (Monthly)

See an experienced Esthetician to care for your skin monthly; the steam, extractions, blending of treatment creams and serums and the massage are all reasons to go see your esthetician every month. Receiving industry free tips and advice from someone who cares for the health of your skin will propel your skincare goals, whether to achieving younger, healthier looking skin.

How to do a self-massage

The muscles in the face need to be toned and firm just as the muscles in the body. Performing daily facial massaging will keep your muscles toned and the skin firm, blood circulating and skin feeling smooth and youthful.

The main idea is to keep stimulating the skin by not only massaging with your hands but by using other tools like the Jade Roller, Gua Sha, High Frequency Wand, the Derma roller and so on. These tools add more efficacy to our products by allowing them to penetrate more effectively in the skin and work. When our skin is stimulated, it functions better, and cells turnover, keeping the skin looking bright and fresh.

As you massage in moisturizers, you start from the inner part of the face, going in an outward and upward motion starting from the cheeks, moving to the forehead in an upward motion, down the temples, down and around the sides of the nose. Sweep around the cheeks, down to the sides of the neck. Then, in an upward motion, stroke your hands up the neck from side to side. As you do, these movements go in quick, firm strokes as you go around the face and neck. Do these 3 or 4 times until the moisturizer has been absorbed.

Chapter 5

Skin Treatment

An inside look into the different skincare treatments

DEEP CLEANSE FACIAL

A Deep Cleanse Facial is one that every skin type and condition will benefit from. It removes dirt, dead cells and impurities, as well as helps to reinvigorate the skin. It is great for men and women of all ages from 13-99. It will keep your skin youthful, hydrated, firm, strong and less prone to breakouts and impurities. The four main skin conditions treated are Acne, Aging, Hyper Pigmentation and Sensitivity. All four will be cleansed, exfoliated, steamed and extracted but treated differently to be healed of its condition.

Below is a list of Facial Treatments.

Grooming deep cleanse

Thanks to coarser skin, larger pores and an increased chance of sun damage, guys need facials probably more than the ladies. Skin damage from your shaving routine or the sun can't be fixed with the soap and water you use every day. Redness fades, but the underlying problems don't get your skin handled by a pro. It will make all the difference.

TEEN DEEP CLEANSE

It's never too early to start your teen on a skincare routine. It's important to begin at an early age to combat conditions such as acne and dry skin. Suitable for 13-19.

SPECIALTY TREATMENTS

DERMAPLANING TREATMENT

Dermaplaning is a cosmetic skin resurfacing procedure and a form of manual exfoliation. This method gently "shaves off "dead skin cells with short strokes and temporarily removes the fine vellus hair (peach fuzz) of the face. The effect is glowing skin with fewer imperfections and a bright silky smooth, even complexion.

Treatment Recommendations: Course of 4-12 treatments every 3-6 weeks

AHA TREATMENT

Glycolic acid is an Alpha-Hydroxy Acid (AHA) derived from sugar cane. It is beneficial for mature, hyper pigmentated or damaged skin and helps to reduce the visible signs of aging. It is especially suitable for dull complexions and smokers' skin with open pores. Glycolic Acid removes dead cells while fighting against skin aging. It increases cellular renewal, stimulates collagen and elastin and therefore reduces the appearance of fine lines. It helps to slow down pigmentation and reduce the dark spots by regulating the melanin synthesis.

Salicylic Acid is a type of Beta hydroxy Acid and comes from the medicinal part of the willow tree called the inner bark. It is for acne-prone skin and helps to reduce the visible acne signs. It is especially recommended for oily skin and helps to remove dead cells while stimulating cellular renewal. Salicylic Acid is an efficient way to improve the epidermis texture, providing an anti-blotching effect. It has real antiseptic and purifying properties which are particularly efficient for acne-prone skin.

Mandelic Acid is an Alpha Hydroxy Acid extracted from bitter almonds. It has proved to be an effective ally for renewing. Thanks to its exfoliating, peeling and delicate action, it soothes and reactivates epidermis cells. It is effective in the treatment against the common cases of skin imperfections such as photo aging, uneven pigmentation and acne. It can be used all year round as there is no risk of hyperpigmentation.

Pumpkin & pomegranate Enzyme Peel is a gentle peel that contains a natural enzyme, Pumpkin, pomegranate Extract, Lactic Acid, Chamomile Extract and Rose Clay. It is suitable for all skin types, including sensitive skin. Enzymes help slough off dead skin cells while moisturizing and rejuvenating the look of the skin, resulting in a healthy, glowing complexion. For best results, it is used with a steamer or warm, wet compresses for 10-15 min, followed by extractions, if needed.

Treatment recommendation: Course of 4-6 treatments or regular individual treatments.

Microneedling treatment

A microneedling treatment will reduce facial scarring, fine lines, hyperpigmentation, sun damage and wrinkles. It will also boost the absorption and concentration of topical skincare products, making them tremendously effective. It can be done for the whole face and neck or in parts, eyes, scars, wrinkles only or just the neck.

Treatment Recommendation: Course of 4-12 treatments every 3-6 weeks.

LED FACIAL THERAPY

LED facial Therapy treatments are relaxing, painless and non-invasive, with multiple benefits. LED treatments work by using an array of bright light-emitting diodes (originally developed by NASA!) that send low-level light energy into the deeper layers of the skin.

LED Therapy is used to help treat various skin conditions such as atopic dermatitis, sensitivity, anti-aging, skin regeneration, acne bacillus, melasma and is great for pain relief (wound healing). There are 7 different colors to treat these conditions as well as combination of conditions to help clear up multiple side effects.

Chapter 6

Key Ingredients

Know Your Ingredients

CHEMICALS THAT HARM

Benzene

Benzene is known to be a carcinogen. Harmful amounts may be absorbed through the skin; it is irritating to the mucous membranes and poisonous when ingested. Because it is usually a trace element, it will not show up on the list of ingredients of cosmetics.

Colors and dyes (FD & C, or D & C)

Artificial colors are made from petroleum and coal tar and are believed to be cancer causing agents. They penetrate the skin, can cause allergies and are irritants to the skin and eyes. They are found on labels as FD & C or D&C and are followed by a color and a number.

DEA (diethanolamine)

This is a synthetic solvent, detergent and humectant widely used in brake fluids, industrial degreasers and antifreeze. It is mostly used in liquid soap, shampoo and conditioner. It can be harmful to the liver, kidney and pancreas. It may cause cancer in various organs. Irritates skin, eyes, and mucous membranes and is a health risk, especially to infants and young children.

Formaldehyde

Due to its bad reputation, it is sometimes hidden under the name DMDM hydantoin or MDM hydantoin. The trade name is Formalin. A common ingredient in shampoos are disinfectants, germicides and fungicides and it is used as a preservative in shampoos. There is a suspected link to some cancers, and it also causes a breakdown of DNA in the skin. Unfortunately, due to the fact that formaldehyde is often used as a preservative in surfactants (washing substances), it is not often listed as an ingredient.

Parabens (methyl, ethyl, propyl, and benzyl)

Cheap preservatives used in beauty-care products that make it possible for them to survive the long trip from China, sit on store or warehouse shelves for years or be exposed to extreme temperatures. When parabens are applied as a cream, the chemicals appear in the blood within hours. Parabens have been shown to mimic estrogen, disrupting our bodies 'endocrine (hormone) system and have been found in human breast tumors possibly linking them to breast cancer. Where possible, use glass containers for your personal beauty products.

Propyl Alcohol (also known as isopropyl alcohol and rubbing alcohol)

Unfortunately, propyl alcohol is not on the list of ingredients as it is used as an antiseptic in the bottling procedure, so theoretically, it is not an ingredient. Traces can be found in most cosmetics, creams, shampoos etc. Possible effects of propyl alcohol include mental depression, headaches and even cancer. The fatal ingested dose is 1 fluid ounce.

Phthalates

Phthalates are industrial chemicals that make plastics soft. They are found in over 70 percent of beauty products and are absorbed through the skin. They have been found to cause birth defects, infertility and other illnesses. If you use plastics, try to transfer the contents to glass containers when possible.

Propylene glycol (common name Antifreeze)

Propylene glycol is the main ingredient in antifreeze, brake and hydraulic fluid. Propylene glycol, the most widely used cosmetic ingredient, is found in moisturizers, baby lotions, makeup, shampoos and hair conditioners. Material safety data sheets on propylene glycol warn users to avoid skin contact as it is systemic and can cause liver abnormalities and kidney damage. Note: it is widely used in baby wipes.

Sodium Lauryl Sulphate and Sodium Laureth Sulphate

Up to 50% of most shampoos are made up of these ingredients. Originally invented to clean garage floors, SLS has been linked to cataracts and cancer. SLS can damage the outer layer of the skin, causing dryness, scaliness, and loss of flexibility. SLS denatures protein and can change genetic material found in cells (mutagenic)

Synthetic Perfumes

Fragrance is used extensively in skin and hair care products and is often the leading cause of allergies and skin problems. Complaints to the FDA concerning perfumes include headaches, dizziness, violent coughing, vomiting and skin irritations and rashes.

Alkyl-phenol ethoxylates

This ingredient is used in the production of shampoo making. Its chemicals mimic estrogen, causing havoc with lowered sperm counts. It has also been linked to breast cancer from the high levels of estrogen. I could write a whole book about dangerous chemicals, but this gives you some idea about what people are using in the commercial marketplace for beauty products.

Ambergris

This is a wax-like substance produced in the intestine of the sperm whale. There is no danger to whales, but it is an animal product.

Gelatin

Used for eye gels. Gelatin is obtained from the bone cartilage of animals.

Lanolin

Lanolin, a purified wax extracted from sheep woo, easily becomes rancid. It does not penetrate the skin, making it useless to use as a carrier for essential oils.

Mineral Oil

Mineral oil is a petroleum by-product. Although it has a long shelf life, which makes it useful as a commercial item, it does not penetrate the skin making it useless for natural skin care.

Petroleum Jelly

Petroleum jelly, a mineral fat, does not penetrate the skin and is also a derivative of crude oil, which is another name for gasoline.

Let's turn now to the ingredients that can contribute to good health and glowing skin.

CHEMICALS THAT HEAL

Algae powder (Laminaria digitata and fucus vesiculosus)

These are powerful detoxifiers and absorb toxins on the skin without harming the living skin. Pure algae becomes active again when it is put into water. It is used in body wraps and as a bath blend. It detoxifies not only the skin but the whole body, making it a wonderful treatment for cellulite and fluid retention.

Carrier oils

A carrier oil is a vegetable oil derived from plants, (from seeds, kernels or nuts). Each carrier oil differs in the therapeutic properties and characteristics that they offer. For example, sesame oil has a sun protection factor of four; jojoba, almond, or apricot kernel oils are true oils, infused oils such as calendula and carrot root (used in many of the recipes in this book) are infused with herbs and roots within a base carrier oil and therefore have additional therapeutic benefits. In choosing carrier oils for use in natural beauty products, choose cold-pressed versions where possible.

Conditioning emulsifier

This is a blend of cetearyl alcohol, castor oil, and stearalkonium chloride. This emulsifying wax improves the ability to detangle the hair and adds shine.

Cornacopa (Chemical name: Decyl polyglucose)

This is made from re-growable raw materials – glucose derived from corn and fatty alcohols from coconut and palm kernel oils. Although cornacopa has been around for years, its use was previously limited by the lack of a large-scale commercial plant. Cornacopa is biodegradable, earth-friendly, orally non-toxic and very mild to the skin and eyes. It can make up to 50% of the shampoo.

Essential oils

Essential oils are extracted by various methods, usually steam distillation from plants, herbs, flowers, trees, seeds and grasses. They have been used in skin and health care for thousands of years and have marvelous therapeutic capabilities. For example, Lavender's delightful and soothing scent also provides antiseptic and analgesic effects. For further reading, the Creamy Craft of Cosmetic Making has a whole chapter devoted to this subject.

Grapefruit seed extract

A by-product of the citrus industry, grapefruit seed extract contains vitamin C and glycerine. Grapefruit seed extract is anti-bacterial, anti-microbial, antiseptic, and can be used internally to combat fungus infections. As a result, this makes a natural preservative for creams, lotions, cosmetics, etc. There are over 600 Lanette waxes on the market, and most that are sold contain sodium lauryl sulphate (see Chemicals that Harm).

Seaweed extract and gel (red algae)

These are extracts from Hypnea Musciformis, Gelidiella Acerosa, Sargassum Filipendula. Seaweed is an antioxidant and is full of easy to absorb proteins, vitamins, minerals and lipids. Repairing and protecting the skin and hair, it reduces oiliness and sebum overproduction and strengthens against damage caused by free radicals.

Wheat protein

This adds protection for the skin and hair as it moisturizes and softens. Wheat protein strengthens the elasticity of the hair and repairs damage to the hair, especially hair that has been overly processed and colored. When added to the shampoo, the wheat protein can make the shampoo into an all-in-one shampoo and conditioner.

Xanthan gum

A gum produced by a pure culture fermentation of a carbohydrate with Xanthomonas campestris, is widely used as a thickener in the cosmetic and food industries.

KEY INGREDIENT-GLOSSARY

ALOE

The humble house plant Aloe Vera is a miracle or wonder plant.

- **Vitamins, enzymes, minerals, carbohydrates, lignin, saponins, salicylic acids,** and amino acids are among the 75 potentially active elements of aloe vera.

It contains antioxidant **vitamins A (beta-carotene), C, and E,** which help to neutralize free radicals. Aloe vera gel has also been reported to protect the skin from UV radiation harm. **Mucopolysaccharides** (sugars in aloe) aid in the retention of moisture in the skin. Aloe stimulates fibroblasts, which create collagen and elastin fibers, resulting in more elastic and wrinkle-free skin.

APRICOT

Apricots are rich in **vitamin E** and **antioxidants**, allowing you to rejuvenate skin cells. The suppler your skin is due to the nourished skin cells, the more radiant your face will be. The best way to benefit from apricots for your facial skin is to apply face creams or masks that contain them.

AVOCADO

Natural oils found in avocados nourish your skin. You can avoid wrinkles, pimples, and blemishes by moisturizing your skin. Avocado is packed with numerous important vitamins and antioxidants that could help nourish your skin from the inside out and give it a natural glow.

BLUEBERRY

Blueberries are **84% water**. They are **nutrient-dense** in addition to being low in calories. They are high in vitamin **C**, **K**, and **manganese**. **Anthocyanins**, which are potent antioxidants that work to reduce the effects of aging, give blueberries their rich blue hue. Blueberries provide many health benefits, including increasing collagen and elastin, decreasing collagen breakdown, brightening, calming and soothing, curing wounds, curing acne, and neutralizing free radicals.

BORAGE SEED OIL

Borage Carrier Oil is thought to reduce inflammation, moisturize and rejuvenate dry skin, treat dermatitis, prevent hair loss, relieve hurting joints, and aid in hormone balance.

CHAMOMILE

Chamomile includes anti-oxidants such as **polyphenols and phytochemicals**. It also contains three compounds, **bisoprolol**, **chamazulene**, and **apigenin**, which provide soothing and healing benefits to sensitive skin. It may help minimize signs of aging by shielding the skin from free radical damage when topically applied to the skin. It promotes cell and **tissue renewal**, which reduces the appearance of fine wrinkles and gives the skin a young glow. Chamomile tea also acts as a **skin bleaching agen**t. It naturally lightens your skin and evens your complexion.

CEDARWOOD

Cedarwood essential oil has **anti-inflammatory**, **antifungal**, and **antibacterial qualities**, making it useful for treating irritated skin as well as acne and eczema. Cedar oil is a strong astringent that is frequently used in natural beauty cleansers since it is effective at eliminating oil.

CRANBERRY

Cranberries are extremely high in polyphenols and vitamins C and E, which effectively fight free radicals to reduce the apparent indications of aging, such as fine lines and wrinkles, hyperpigmentation, and loss of elasticity.

CYPRESS

Cypress oil helps to **restore skin hydration** and soothes oily and dry skin. Cypress oil is also a **natural astringent**, which can help reduce the look of oil on the skin without over-drying it. Cypress oil's **decongestant properties** help to minimize skin discoloration and puffiness. **Skin-soothing qualities** soothe irritated and inflamed skin and hasten recovery.

CARROT SEED

The carrot seed oil has;

- **Detoxifying qualities**
- **Antibacterial properties.**
- **Anti-fungal properties.**

This oil aids in the prevention of skin allergies, the reduction of inflammation, and the restoration of damaged skin. It also aids in the prevention of acne outbreaks and congested pores. Carrot seed oil on the face relaxes the skin by reducing redness, irritation, acne, and scars. By removing these, you can maintain your skin calm and clear.

CAYENNE

Cayenne pepper contains capsaicin, which is a powerful anti-inflammatory, making it ideal for puffy, aged skin. It also energizes the skin by increasing blood flow to the area. Cayenne is ideal for treating acne and acne scars due to its **high vitamin** and **antioxidant content** and **calming anti-inflammatory**, **anti-fungal, anti-allergen**, and **anti-irritant characteristics.**

COCONUT

Coconut oil has **anti-inflammatory characteristics** that make it useful for irritated, chafed skin. Coconut oil contains **lauric acid**, which **promotes collagen formation**. Collagen aids in the maintenance of skin firmness and suppleness.

CALENDULA

Calendula oil has **antifungal, anti-inflammatory,** and **antibacterial qualities**, making it excellent for wound healing, eczema relief, and diaper rash relief. Its qualities are acknowledged by the WHO and are usually deemed safe for use on the skin.

COQ10

CoQ10, also known as **Coenzyme Q10**, has antioxidant characteristics that protect the skin from environmental stresses, energize the skin, and aid in moisture retention. It helps equal skin tone, reduces dullness, and tightens the skin.

DANDELION

Dandelion detoxifies the skin, clears pores, clears acne, and prevents future outbreaks as an antibacterial, germicide, and anti-fungal component. It's difficult to discover a solution that works for both acne-prone skin and a variety of other skin types, but the dandelion is a true wonder worker in this regard.

EVENING PRIMROSE

Evening primrose oil has high levels of **omega-6 polyunsaturated fatty acids**. These chemicals have strong **anti-inflammatory characteristics**, which may aid in treating and preventing acne. Evening primrose oil has emollient characteristics in skincare formulas, which means it softens and smoothens the skin, enhancing its overall texture.

FENNEL

All skin types benefit greatly from fennel, especially oily and acne-prone skin. The bacteria and filth that cause oil accumulation and breakouts are eliminated by its antiseptic capabilities. Acne treatment using fennel compounds like limonene, anethole, and myrcene is so lit in the skin care industry.

FRANKINCENSE

Strong astringent properties of frankincense essential oil aid in protecting skin cells. It can help fade acne scars, hide enlarged pores, avoid wrinkles, and even lift and tighten skin to help naturally halt aging.

GERANIUM

Geranium oil is a great **antioxidant, antimicrobial** and **anti-inflammatory oil** that actively improves the health and natural radiance of the skin. It protects skin from harsh weather conditions and acne by keeping it conditioned and soothing irritated or breakout-prone skin.

GLYCERIN

Glycerin is beneficial to the skin because it functions as a **humectant**, a substance that assists the skin in retaining moisture. It can help to hydrate the skin, reduce dryness, and renew the skin's surface. It's also an **emollient**, meaning it can soften skin.

GRAPESEED

Grape seed extract increases **cell turnover** and **collagen formation**, allowing your skin to remain supple and healthy. Because of the **antioxidants** and **microbiological qualities**, skincare and beauty products using grape seed extract help improve your face tone and treat acne outbreaks when used regularly.

GRAPEFRUIT

Beta Carotene, a powerful antioxidant, improves dull, dry complexions and gives your skin a gorgeous, vibrant glow. Additionally, **Lycopene,** which is believed to lessen skin irritation and redness and assist in balancing out skin tone for a flawless complexion, is found in grapefruit.

GREEN TEA

The anti-inflammatory effects of green tea can help lessen swelling, redness, and skin irritation. Green tea can also be used to treat sunburns and minor wounds. Studies have discovered that topical green tea is an effective treatment for numerous dermatological diseases because of its anti-inflammatory qualities.

GOTU KOLA

Gotu kola is well-known for its ability to promote blood flow, hence assisting the skin's healing process. It reduces pimples, scars, and blemishes and is useful in treating varicose veins, broken capillaries, and persistent cellulite.

HAZELNUT

Oleic acid, a fatty acid that contributes to skin moisturization and maintains the skin looking visibly moisturized, is abundant in hazelnut oil. Because it contains many fatty acids and vitamin E, hazelnut oil is well known for its ability to hydrate. Vitamin E can keep your skin looking smooth and silky.

HORSETAIL

Horsetail Extract exfoliates the skin, reduces the visibility of big pores, and encourages firmer, tauter skin. It also delivers **anti-aging effects**, increases collagen formation, reduces the appearance of wrinkles and fine lines, and shields against free radicals. Horsetail also accelerates the healing process to treat burns, cuts, and wounds.

HYALURONIC ACID

Hyaluronic acid allows the skin to stretch and flex while also reducing wrinkles and creases. Hyaluronic acid has also been shown to help wounds heal faster and minimize scarring. It is safe and useful to use on a daily basis to keep skin hydrated.

HIBISCUS

Hibiscus improves the skin's capacity to retain moisture, which is essential for maintaining a young appearance. Its naturally moisturizing properties keep skin hydrated, soft, and supple for longer, preventing dry, dull skin.

HEMPSEED

Hemp seed oil is **abundant in antioxidants**, including vitamins **A, C, E, and F**, as well as **fatty acids**, which help to build the skin's outer layer and allow it to retain water. This keeps the skin tighter and decreases the appearance of fine lines and wrinkles.

HONEY

Honey is a humectant, which means it absorbs and retains moisture, keeping your skin from drying out. It is also very soothing to the skin. Honey contains natural antioxidants and anti-microbial qualities that protect, heal, and prevent skin damage.

JUNIPER

Antibacterial, antiseptic, and **anti-inflammatory** effects are found in juniper berries. These properties aid in the treatment of acne and outbreaks. They also aid in balancing the skin's sebum production by lowering excess oil production. This decreases pore clogging and blocking, leading to acne and outbreaks.

JOJOBA

Jojoba oil balances natural oil production while hydrating, softening, and smoothing the skin. It provides antioxidant protection and may aid in acne reduction.

LEMONGRASS

Lemongrass oil improves overall skin texture by cleansing and detoxifying the skin and pores and removing excess oil. The oil's **antioxidant capabilities** aid in the neutralization of free radicals and the promotion of skin suppleness.

LAVENDER

Lavender oil hydrates the skin softly and is non-comedogenic. Lavender oil is naturally **antimicrobial**, which eliminates acne-causing germs that may invade your pores. As a result, it is ideal for preventing, soothing, and curing severe acne breakouts.

LEMON

Because lemons are high in **vitamin C** and **citric acid**, they can help brighten and lighten your skin over time. Vitamin C is an excellent antioxidant for fighting free radicals and increasing collagen formation. That is, it can aid in the lightening of black patches.

LICORICE

Licorice contains **glycyrrhizin**, which helps reduce redness, irritation, and swelling and treats skin disorders such as atopic dermatitis and eczema. Licorice helps in calming skin and reduces inflammation.

MYRRH

Myrrh Essential Oil helps to fade undesirable blemishes on the skin, calms irritation and lowers eczema symptoms, among other skin disorders. It cleans, hydrates, and tightens the skin, minimizing and preventing more chapping and sagging.

MACADAMIA NUT

Macadamia nut oil is high in monounsaturated fats and a good source of Vitamin E, making it easy to absorb without leaving your skin feeling greasy. These fatty acids nourish the skin, aid in treating dry skin and help retain moisture. It mimics your skin's natural oils, helping keep your natural radiance.

MSM

MSM can help promote collagen and prevent wrinkles and creases when applied to the face. It also increases **keratin**, another protein that contributes to the stiffness of your skin and aids in the protective barrier of your skin.

NEROLI

Neroli Essential Oil has strong antibacterial characteristics, making it an excellent element for treating acne and balancing sebum production. It fights free radicals and soothes breakout-induced irritation and redness because it is high in antioxidants.

OAT

Oatmeal can absorb extra oil from your skin and aid in acne treatment. **Saponins**, which are natural cleaners, are also found in oats. Its **antioxidant and anti-inflammatory characteristics** aid in treating dry skin and removing dead skin cells.

OLIVE OIL

Olive oil contains antioxidants and flavonoids, which protect the skin from sun damage, dust, and pollution. It's a fantastic moisturizer for dry skin. Olive oil reduces oil production and cleans and unclogs pores in oily skin.

PAPAYA

Papaya is extremely beneficial in treating dry skin and hydrating your skin. Papaya's high concentration of antioxidants and enzymes aids in treating dry and flaky skin.

PUMPKIN

You know, pumpkin has the highest naturally occurring **vitamin A** content, which helps lessen acne scars; **salicylic acid**, which helps reduce acne; and **beta carotene**, which helps decrease wrinkles & dark spots. Furthermore, its high zinc concentration protects your skin against UV radiation.

POMEGRANATE

Pomegranate for skin is high in vitamin C, which has been shown in studies to be useful in healing dull and dry skin. It can minimize skin roughness when used topically regularly.

PUMICE

When lava and water combine, a pumice stone forms. It's a lightweight yet abrasive stone for removing dry, dead skin. A pumice stone can also soften calluses and corns, reducing friction pain.

ROSEMARY

Rosemary Oil is a pleasant **astringent** that tones and balances the skin complexion. When applied topically, it helps to decongest acne and oily skin types while maintaining skin balance.

ROSEHIP

Rosehip oil is high in **vitamins A, C**, and **E** and **vital fatty acids**. These fatty acids are antimicrobial and can help with aging, pigmentation, and skin hydration.

RHUBARB

Rhubarb has **antifungal** and **antibacterial** properties. Raw rhubarb paste has frequently been used as a topical therapy for numerous skin infections like acne.

ROSE GERANIUM

Skincare experts believe that rose geranium regulates the skin's normal oil production, reduces the appearance of enlarged pores, gets rid of microorganisms that cause infections or acne, and improves circulation.

TEA TREE

Because of its anti-inflammatory and antibacterial characteristics, tea tree oil is a popular acne treatment. It is said to reduce redness, edema, and inflammation. It may even aid in preventing and reducing acne scarring, leaving you with smooth, clear skin.

TAMANU

Tamanu aids in the production of collagen and other skin-care components. It can also help minimize scars in addition to mending wounds. Minor burns and sunburns are soothed. Tamanu oil is frequently used to treat sunburns and mild burns.

TURMERIC

Turmeric includes antioxidants as well as anti-inflammatory properties. These features may give the skin a glow and sparkle. Turmeric may also revitalize your skin by enhancing its natural glow.

SWEET ALMOND OIL

Almond oil is high in vitamin D, vitamin E (Tocopherol), and minerals, which help relieve inflammation, protect against UV radiation damage and replenish the skin's moisture barrier.

SEA BUCKTHORN

The berries of the Sea Buckthorn plant have up to 12 times the Vitamin C content of oranges! Because of this, it is excellent for brightening the complexion and leveling out any pigmentation or age spots. It can act as a moisturizing ingredient since it includes linoleic acid, which is naturally found in sebum and may assist in regulating moisture levels and overall hydration.

SAFFLOWER OIL

Safflower oil is **non-comedogenic**, which means it does not clog pores. Its **anti-inflammatory properties** may also be beneficial in treating pimples and acne patches. Using it a few times per week may also help cleanse your pores.

SUGAR CANE

Sugarcane juice is the most effective way to treat any skin problems. It contains many acids like **glycolic** and **alpha-hydroxy (AHA)**, which boost cell formation. They also aid in exfoliating the skin and reducing the likelihood of acne formation. Sugarcane juice is high in minerals such as calcium and phosphorus.

SANDALWOOD

Sandalwood oil nourishes the skin, improves cell suppleness, and evens skin tone. Because of these characteristics, it may be useful in reducing the appearance of scars.

SUNFLOWER OIL

Sunflower oil contains **antioxidants** that help prevent premature aging and wrinkles, keeping your skin appearing young and fresh. Sunflower oil also has **linoleic acid**, which aids in the retention of moisture in the skin, making it less dry.

SWEET ORANGE

Orange Essential Oil benefits skin health, look, and texture by increasing clarity, shine, and smoothness, decreasing the indications of acne and other unpleasant skin disorders.

SHEA BUTTER

Shea butter acts as an emollient. It may soften or smooth dry skin. Shea butter also contains anti-inflammatory properties. This could aid in treating skin disorders related to swelling, such as eczema.

VITAMIN C

This amazing antioxidant and anti-inflammatory ingredient have been shown to improve skin tone and texture, moisturize the skin, and minimize indications of aging. Including vitamin C in your skincare routine will not only brighten your complexion but also prevent it from sun damage and damaging free radicals.

VITAMIN A

Vitamin A supports natural moisturizing, which means it helps to hydrate the skin effectively, giving it a bright glow. It also helps speed healing, reduce breakouts, and boost the skin's immune system. It aids in the promotion and maintenance of a healthy dermis and epidermis, or the top two layers of your skin.

VITAMIN B3

Vitamin B3, in its niacinamide form, prevents water loss and keeps the skin's moisture content. It has also been shown to boost keratin. Regarding aging skin, niacinamide enhances the surface structure, smoothing out the texture and reducing the appearance of wrinkles.

VITAMIN B5

Pro-Vitamin B5 aids in the maintenance of soft, smooth, and healthy skin. It also has an anti-inflammatory impact, which can aid in your skin's healing processes. It is deeply moisturizing and helps to keep skin hydrated by absorbing moisture from the air.

VITAMIN E

Vitamin E is best known for its skin health and beauty advantages. Topically applied to the face, it can relieve inflammation and rejuvenate the skin.

WITCH HAZEL

Tannins are compounds found in witch hazel. Witch hazel, when applied directly to the skin, may help reduce swelling, mend injured skin, and combat bacteria.

WHEAT GERM

Wheat Germ Carrier Oil moisturizes and protects the skin while softening and increasing skin flexibility. The oil contains anti-aging compounds that help the skin diminish outward indications of age, like wrinkles. The oil has several emollient characteristics that help to soothe dry skin.

WILLOW BARK

Willow bark extract is an effective herbal treatment for various skin issues. It exfoliates your skin, reduces excess oil, clears your pores, and keeps your skin hydrated.

Chapter 7

Skin & Diet

Green Smoothie Diet & Benefits

The Secret to Vibrant, Radiant Health

A healthy body is vibrant and full of energy and life. Natural, healthy eating is the secret to inner and outer beauty. When eating natural, raw foods, you simply look and feel better and younger. Once you eat in a manner that keeps your cells clean and healthy, you will begin to look radiant despite your age.

Human beings are designed to eat a diet primarily made up of fruits, vegetables, seeds and nuts. With these types of natural, healthy foods, our bodies flourish and receive all of the necessary nutrients to keep our bodies toxin-free and looking our most beautiful.

One of the first places where you'll see changes is in the quality of your skin. Healthy eating and living will remove years from your face, eliminate wrinkles, fade age spots and give you a "second youth." Your skin will become supple, and acne will clear up. Your eyes will become brighter and begin to sparkle. The dark circles and puffiness will diminish, as will the yellowness in the whites of your eyes. On the inside of your body, your cells will become rejuvenated as well, causing your organs to function more efficiently.

Take control of your health by caring for your body and feeding it what it needs to be radiant, healthy and vibrant. What makes us feel old is sludge and waste that gets trapped in the body. Anti-aging creams and cosmetic surgery won't clean that out. Your skin will look more youthful because your cells will become tighter and healthier as you hydrate and detox the body.

BENEFITS OF THE GREEN SMOOTHIES

Green Smoothies will give your body the quality nutrition it needs while cleansing your cells and insides. Vitamins, minerals and other nutrients will be absorbed by your body more efficiently, allowing your cells to become like new as you begin to look and feel younger. Green Smoothies are very simple. They consist of raw organic fruit, raw organic leafy greens and water and the recommended fruit: greens ratio is 6:4, so you're getting the right amount of nutrients to feed your body. They are filling and healthy, and your body will thank you for drinking them.

Despite their simplicity, green smoothies provide a ton of nutritional benefits that lead to a healthier lifestyle. These benefits include:

- weight loss
- increased energy
- reduction in food cravings
- clearer skin
- nutrient - rich
- detoxifying
- vibrant, radiant health
- improved digestion
- hydration

Once you try out these recipes, you'll discover that there are many other benefits for yourself. Stay consistent and have this regimen be a part of your lifestyle.

WHICH GREENS & WHY

Here is a list of green leafy vegetables that are most popular to use in the nutrient-rich Green Smoothies.

Arugula: Arugula is a great source of folic acid as well as vitamins A, C, and K, and provides a boost for bone and brain health. It has a zippy, peppery flavor.

Beet Greens: Beet greens are the leafy tops of the beet vegetable. They are rich in vitamin K. They are known to help improve vision, help prevent Alzheimer's, and boost the immune system.

Bok Choy: Bok choy is a Chinese cabbage that is mild-tasting and crunchy. It is full of vitamins A, C, and calcium, as well as antioxidants.

Chard (aka Swiss Chard): Chard is a green leafy vegetable that displays red stalks, leaf veins, and stems. It has a beet-like taste and a mild texture. It is known to help prevent cancers and is good for cleansing the digestive system.

Collard Greens: Collards are green leafy vegetables that are nutritionally similar to kale but chewier and with a much stronger taste. They are a superior agent for binding to bile acids throughout the digestive tract, which makes them very good at lowering cholesterol.

Dandelion Greens: Dandelion greens look like weeds in your lawn, but they are yet another great source of vitamins A and K. They help the digestion process and can help constipation issues because they are a natural laxative.

Kale: Kale is lightweight with ruffled leaf edges. It is loaded with vitamins A, C, K, and more. It is known for lowering the risks associated with developing prostate, ovary, breast, colon, and bladder cancers.

Lettuce: Lettuce has been a popular staple in salads since the time of the Ancient Egyptians. It contains essential amino acids and vitamins. Be sure to eat lettuce with dark green leaves to get the highest nutritional value. Romaine lettuce, in particular, has high levels of vitamins C, K, and A is a good source of folic acid.

Mustard Greens: Spicy mustard greens are effective in lowering cholesterol and provide a healthy dose of riboflavin, niacin, magnesium, and iron. They are a storehouse of phytonutrients that have many disease-preventing properties.

Parsley: Parsley is rich in antioxidants, minerals, vitamins, and fiber and is known to help reduce aging and regulate blood sugar levels.

Spinach: Perhaps the most beloved green leafy vegetable of them all, spinach is mild tasting and not as bitter as other greens. Its dark green leaves really pack a punch with high levels of omega-3s, calcium, magnesium, and vitamins A, C, E, and K. When most people start drinking green smoothies, they start with spinach!

Turnip Greens: Turnip greens, although slightly bitter, are very flavorful. Turnip greens are effective at providing numerous health benefits, but they stand out amongst other green leafy veggies in their ability to fight the development of cancerous cells.

Milder-Tasting Greens:

- Baby beet greens
- Baby bok choy
- Butter lettuce
- Carrot top greens
- Kale
- Romaine lettuce
- Spinach
- Swiss chard
- *Stronger-Tasting Greens:*
- Arugula
- Collard greens
- Dandelion greens
- Mustard greens
- Radish tops
- Sorrel
- Turnip greens
- Watercress

Darker varieties of green leafy vegetables provide chlorophyll and other very important nutrients. Some examples of dark, leafy greens are chard, spinach, kale, baby salad greens, arugula, romaine lettuce, dandelion greens, beet greens and collard greens. Always remember organic produce is superior.

GREEN SMOOTHIE RECIPES FOR BEAUTY & ANTI-AGEING

Blending Instruction: Place the leafy greens and whatever liquids are called for (or ice) into the blender and blend until the mixture has a juice-like consistency. Stop the blender and add the remaining ingredients. Blend until creamy. Add protein powder and other seeds like flax, chia and/or hemp seeds to the mix for added benefit. Instead of stevia, feel free to substitute for raw organic honey.

Peach Banana Greens

- 2 handfuls greens
- 2 cups water
- 1 1/2 cups frozen peaches
- 1 banana, peeled
- 2 tablespoons sunflower oil
- 2 teaspoons spirulina

Berry Coconut

- 2 handfuls greens
- 1 1/2 cups coconut water
- 1/2 cup frozen blueberries
- 1/2 cup frozen raspberries

Watermelon Ginger Greens

- 2 handfuls greens
- 1/2 cup ice
- 4 cups watermelon chunks
- 2 tablespoons chia seeds
- 1 inch fresh ginger, peeled

Banana Nut Greens

- 2 handfuls greens
- 1 1/2 cups almond milk
- 3 bananas, peeled
- 2 tablespoons chia seeds

Mango Banana

- 2 handfuls greens
- 1 cup coconut water
- 1 banana, peeled
- 1 1/2 cups frozen mango chunks

Papaya Lemon

- 1 handful parsley
- 2 cups water
- 1 banana, peeled and frozen
- 1 cup papaya chunks

- 1 lemon

Orange Spinach

- 2 cups baby spinach
- 1 orange, peeled and seeded
- 1 kiwi, peeled
- 1 tablespoon apple cider vinegar
- 1 packet stevia

Banana Pear

- 2 handfuls greens
- 1 1/2 cups water
- 1 banana, peeled and frozen
- 2 pears
- 1/3 cup almond butter

Apple Pear

- 2 handfuls greens
- 2 stalks celery, chopped
- 1/2 cup water
- 1 pear, seeded
- 1 large apple
- 1 banana, peeled and frozen
- 2 tablespoons fresh lemon juice

Green Berry

- 2 handfuls greens
- 1/2 cup water
- 1/2 cup green tea
- 2 cups mixed berries
- 1 banana, peeled and frozen

Carrot Apple

- 2 handfuls greens
- 3 stalks celery
- 1 cup water
- 1 small beet, peeled and diced
- 1 cup ice
- 2 carrots
- 1 apple
- 1/2 lemon, seeded, peeled, and sectioned

Cranberry Berry

- 2 handfuls greens
- 1/2 cup ice
- 1/2 cup blueberries
- 1/2 cup blackberries
- 1/2 cup cranberries

- 1 tablespoon ground chia seeds

Cucumber Strawberry

- 2 handfuls greens
- 1 cup water
- 1 cucumber
- 1 cup frozen strawberries
- 4 dried figs
- 2 tablespoons ground flaxseeds

* 9 7 9 8 8 6 4 9 0 8 5 9 4 *